How To Grow Taller Naturally

HTeBooks

Copyright © 2016

Disclaimer

This book is designed to provide condensed information. It is not intended to reprint all the information that is otherwise available, but instead to complement, amplify and supplement other texts. You are urged to read all the available material, learn as much as possible and tailor the information to your individual needs.

Every effort has been made to make this book as complete and as accurate as possible. However, there may be mistakes, both typographical and in content. Therefore, this text should be used only as a general guide and not as the ultimate source of information. The purpose of this book is to educate.

The author or the publisher shall have neither liability nor responsibility to any person or entity with respect to any loss or damage caused, or alleged to have been caused, directly or indirectly, by the information contained in this book.

Table of Contents

How Will This Book Help You?

There is no doubt that being tall has its advantages. It is always ideal for us to achieve our maximum height potential so that we can cash in on its benefits. But when we talk about growing taller, many people start to think of acupressure treatments, medications, and other external alternatives without realizing that there are natural methods we can do to help us grow taller.

In this book, you will learn how eating the right kinds of food, exercising on a regular basis, having proper posture and adequate sleep can effectively help you reach your maximum height potential. You will also learn the things that you need to avoid in order to prevent stunted growth. The good news is that the techniques you will learn in this book will not only help you become taller but they can also help you achieve a healthier and fitter body.

Eat the Right Kinds of Food

"The food you eat can be either the safest and most powerful form of medicine or the slowest form of poison."

- Ann Wigmore

Our height is primarily determined by our genes but it can also greatly depend on the food that we eat, particularly during the growing years. If we eat the right kinds of food, we can expect to reach our maximum height. On the other hand, if we are deprived of certain nutrients, our growth may become stunted. The main nutrient that enables the body to grow is protein which is considered as the building block for our skeletal system including the tissues, cartilages and bones. Our skeletal system provides the frame for our body wherein the mass composed of fat and muscles are added to.

It is therefore essential that we eat adequate amounts of protein during our formative years to ensure that we reach our maximum height potential. But as we try to increase our consumption of protein-enriched foods, we need to be cautious in consuming foods that contain a lot of carbohydrates and fats. Too much carbs and fats can actually hinder the metabolism of proteins and as a result deter the growth rate.

Some of the protein-enriched foods that you can include in your regular diet are: oatmeal, skimmed milk, soybeans, eggs, meat and poultry. It is also ideal that your regular food diet includes other food groups that aid in developing your entire body. Make sure that you eat enough meat, fruits, vegetables, grains and good fats. Always go for high quality foods to ensure that you are not taking in toxins and other harmful ingredients that can hamper your growth. It is also ideal to increase your calcium intake since calcium is very vital in the growth of the bones. But in order for the calcium to be absorbed by your body, you need to ensure that you are getting sufficient vitamin D.

Importance of Vitamins

Vitamins are among the most critical factors in ensuring maximum height growth and for sustaining a healthy body. Of all the vitamins that we need to intake, Vitamin D can be considered as one of the most essential not only for promoting maximum growth but for proper maintenance of strong bones, as well. As such, if you wish to reach your maximum height, it is vital that you eat vitamin D enriched foods on a regular basis. Some of the foods rich in vitamin D include cauliflower, potatoes, tomatoes and other citrus fruits. By eating these foods on a regular basis, you will prevent vitamin deficiencies that can result to stunted growth.

Another essential vitamin that you need to take to ensure maximum growth is Vitamin B1. Some of the foods that are rich in Vitamin B1 are peanuts, rice, pork, beans and soybeans. Vitamin B1 does not only aid in enhancing growth but in ensuring proper functioning of the cardiovascular, digestion and nervous systems.

Vitamin B2, referred to as riboflavin, is also essential in ensuring maximum height growth. You can get it from foods such as fish, eggs, green leafy vegetables and milk.

You should also ensure that you have sufficient levels of Vitamin C to ensure that your bones and muscles will grow in a healthy manner. You can get Vitamin C from tomatoes, berries, potatoes and most citrus fruits.

Importance of Zinc and Minerals

Aside from vitamin-enriched foods, you also need to include foods rich in zinc and other minerals in your regular food diet in order to grow up to your maximum height potential. The most essential minerals that you should prevent becoming deficient from include zinc, fluoride, calcium, iodine and manganese. Calcium helps in developing and sustaining strong bones and it can be commonly be found in dairy products, especially milk.

Foods that are rich in minerals include collards, turnips, spinach and most soy food products. Research studies have shown that increased consumption of zinc-enriched foods can actually aid in increasing height. Some of the zinc-enriched foods include yeast, eggs, peanuts, lamb, dried watermelon seeds, steak, pumpkin seeds and oysters. Zinc is not only essential in ensuring maximum growth but it is also very useful in enhancing the metabolism of the body.

Iodine is another essential mineral that helps in boosting growth. By ensuring that you have adequate supply of iodine in your body, you will not only ensure maximum growth but you can also ensure that your thyroid gland is functioning properly and the rest of your body parts are developing properly. Some of the iodine-enriched foods include fish, cereals, meat, tomatoes and green peas.

Do you need to take supplements in order to increase height?

As discussed above, you need to ensure that you have sufficient amounts of proteins, fats, carbohydrates, minerals and vitamins in your regular diet in order to ensure maximum growth. But many people find it difficult to get or prepare foods that contain the recommended daily allowance for each of the essential nutrients. This is the reason why diet supplements have been made available in the market. However, before you decide to buy and consume food supplements, you should consult your doctor to ensure that you will not be taking in supplements that can only bring harm instead of benefits. There are certain hormonal supplements and medications that aid in activating the body's growth glands. When taken properly or as prescribed, these supplements promise to increase your height by a couple of inches. But you do not really need those ultra-advanced supplements. You just need to ensure that you have sufficient supply of calcium and Vitamin D in your regular diet – either through natural foods or supplements. Many people forget to boost their Vitamin D which makes their calcium intake ineffective.

*)Grow up to your maximum height potential by nourishing your body with sufficient amounts of the essential nutrients that it needs.

Get Into a Regular Exercise Routine

"To enjoy the glow of good health, you must exercise."

- Gene Tunney

Without a doubt, height can play a vital role in improving a person's identity. This is the reason why a lot of people look for ways to enhance their height in any possible manner. Because of increasing demand, we can now see a lot of different acupressure treatments and other medications that declare their effectiveness in increasing a person's height. However, before you shell out your hard earned money to purchase these very expensive treatments, you need to spend enough time in assessing their validity. You need to be aware of the harmful side effects that these treatments normally have. You would not want to risk your health for treatments that cannot really guarantee 100% effectiveness.

Before you look for artificial treatments to increase your height, it is ideal for you to first seek natural methods such as regular exercise regimes combined with proper diet and nutrition. With proper physical exercise, you will not only increase your chances of growing up to your fullest height potential but you will also be able to tone and strengthen your muscles and sustain a healthy and fit body. Just remember to always combine physical exercise with proper diet in order to maintain active and fresh growth hormones and to repair and build your muscles.

Even though it is a widely accepted fact that our height is primarily influenced by our genes, we can still do certain things such as exercise and diet to improve our chances of reaching our fullest height potential. Typically, we stop growing after the start of adolescence because of the merging of the growth plates in the long bones in the body. However, it is always possible for you to continue growing and add a couple of inches even when you are in your early 20's by doing specific exercise routines that boost growth in height.

To achieve the optimum results, you can adopt and practice the following exercises two to three times per week. Just make sure that you do not over-exercise because doing so will only lead to injuries that can ultimately lead to stunted growth.

Bar Hanging

Did you know that gravity can actually make you look shorter because it compresses your joints and spines which eventually thins and squeezes the cartilage? One of the best and simplest ways to fight this problem is by hanging from a vertical bar. When you hang from a bar, you allow the weight of your lower torso to elongate your spine and decrease the pull on your vertebra. This can then result to increased height by about one to two inches. But do not think that the height increase will happen after only one exercise. You need to be patient and perform this exercise on a regular basis.

The horizontal bar that you will use for this exercise must be positioned at a height where you can let your body to extend with sufficient room to move. If it is not possible for you to have a bar that will allow your body to completely extend, you can simply slightly bend both of your knees so that you will still hang without restrictions. Make sure that you are securely gripping the bar and that the palms of your hands are outward facing. While you are hanging on the bar, make sure that your shoulders, arms and hips are kept as relaxed as possible. This will allow gravity to really pull your body downwards. To add an extra pull, you can opt to wear ankle weights.

You should freely hang on the bar for around twenty seconds. Then take a rest before repeating for at least three to four times. Amongst the exercises known to increase height, bar hanging is considered to be the most effective.

Dry Land Swim

Dry land swimming is also commonly referred to as alternate kicking. The focus of this exercise is your lower back.

To begin the exercise, lie down with your stomach flat on a mat or the floor. Make sure that your entire body is completely extended. Put both of your arms in front of you. Make sure that the palms of your hand are facing downwards toward the floor. Slowly raise your right arm higher than the left arm. Make sure that both your legs are completely straight. As you do so, lift your left leg as high off the floor as you can. Stay in this position for a minimum of four seconds. Then do the same steps with your left arm and right leg. Your objective is to eventually sustain this position for at least 20 seconds.

If you want to increase the benefits of this exercise, you can put on ankle and wrist weights which can increase the resistance and tone the muscles on your lower back.

Pelvic Shift

Despite the extreme simplicity of this exercise, it is very effective in giving your body a good up and down stretch from both your hips and spine.

To begin the exercise, lie down with your back on the mat or floor. Put your arms and shoulders firmly on the mat. Then bend both of your knees and keep both of your feet as close to your butt as possible. The next step is to arch your back so you can thrust your pelvis in an upward position. Keep this position for around twenty to thirty seconds. By regularly doing this exercise, you will be able to stretch and make your front hips more flexible.

Cobra Stretch

The objective of this yoga exercise is to give your spine a good stretch which can then make it more flexible and supple. This specific exercise is very effective in allowing the cartilages in between your vertebra to grow. The ultimate result is increased height.

To do this exercise, lie down on a mat or floor with your face downwards and the palms of both your arms on floor right under the shoulders. Completely arch your spine until your chin has come to its highest angle. You can arch as far as you can but each time you try this exercise, aim to arch back farther. Do this exercise for a minimum of three to four repetitions. Hold the position for five to thirty seconds before resting.

Super Cobra Stretch

To do this exercise, lie down on a mat or floor with your face downwards and the palms of both your arms on floor right under the shoulders. Completely arch your spine until your chin has come to its highest angle. Then bend your hips so you can make your body get into an upturned V position. As you do the stretch, make sure that your chin is firmly tucked against your chest. Hold the position for ten to twenty seconds and then go back to the original position and rest.

Hopping with One Leg

This is another super simple exercise that you can do just about anywhere. You can do this exercise while you are watching your favorite TV show or you are watching your kids play in the park or while you are doing your other household chores.

Simply hop on your right leg 8 times while keeping your hands pointed upwards. Afterwards, then do the same thing on your left leg. The bouncing motion is good not only in activating your growth hormones but in developing your brain and strengthening your legs, as well.

Pilates Roll Over

This is a superb exercise that can help in giving your spine a good stretch. It can also give your upper body extra length. Another good benefit of doing this exercise is that the vertebra in your neck area will also be stretched and lengthened.

To do begin this exercise, lie on a mat or on the floor with your back on the floor and your arms resting on your sides. Make sure that the palms of your hands are facing down. Keep both of your legs together and then lengthen them until they are straight and pointing upwards to the ceiling. Then bend your legs backwards so that they touch the mat. You may think that touching the mat or the floor in this position may seem hard at first. But be assured that as you continue to practice this exercise, it will become easier. Always keep in mind that the more you perform stretching exercises, the more your spine will become lengthened and flexible.

Forward Spine Stretch

To begin this exercise, sit on a mat with your back straight and your feet straight in front of you. Make sure that both of your legs are extended out. Your legs should also be apart with at least shoulder width. As you breathe in, extend both of your arms in front. And as you breathe, slowly bend forward and continue to stretch your arms until you can reach your toes. When you stretch forward this way, you are making your spine become flexed at its maximum limit. If you are not flexible enough to reach your toes, it is alright. Just try to reach as far forward as you can. As you continue to practice your flexibility exercises, your body will become suppler.

Cat Stretch

This flexibility exercise is also referred to as the Indian Dandwat. The objective of this exercise is to help in opening up your spine while strengthening your back, shoulders, palms and chest. While you perform this exercise, you will be stretching your hamstrings while placing stress on your stomach area.This exercise is also very helpful in improving blood circulation.

To begin this exercise, put your knees and hands on a mat or on the floor. Make sure that both of your arms are locked out. Breathe in while you flex your spine down and then breathe out while you arch your back and bring your head down. At this point, arch your spine as far up as you can while keeping your elbows straight and your shoulders high. Make sure that at this position, your pelvic bone is touching the floor. Repeat the cycle for 10 to 12 times with each cycle lasting three to eight seconds.

The Bow Down

To begin this exercise, stand up straight while placing both of your hands on the hips. While you stay in this standing position, slowly bend forwards as far as you can. Make sure that your head is leading the bend. But keep in mind that your knees should be straight or locked. While bent down, make sure that your chin is not touching your chest. Repeat this cycle for 3 to 5 times with each cycle lasting for four to eight seconds.

Forward Bend

This is another very popular and commonly followed stretching exercise that is known to help in increasing height. To begin this exercise, stand up straight while keeping your legs wide apart. While you are in this position, extend up your hands keeping it straight. Then slowly bend forward until you are touching the floor with your hands. But make sure that your knees are not bended. After 3 seconds, go back to the first position.

Spot Jump

To begin this exercise, stand up straight while keeping both of your legs closed. Then slowly lift your body until you are standing on your toes. Then begin jumping with your hands straightened up. Continue jumping for a minimum of two minutes.

Hands on the Head Bow Down

To begin this exercise, stand up while placing both of your hands at the back of your neck. Then slowly bend forward as far down as you can. Bend down until your chin is touching your chest but make sure that your knees are not bent. Repeat the cycle for 3 to 5 times with each cycle lasting for four to eight seconds. If you cannot touch your chest yet, just be patient. Just keep in mind that your flexibility will improve as you continuously practice the exercises.

Super Stretch

To begin this exercise, stand up while placing both of your hands at the back of your neck. Then slowly bend your head backwards as far down as you can. Repeat the cycle for 3 to 5 times with each cycle lasting for five to fifteen seconds.

Wall Stretch

To begin this exercise, stand up with your back against a wall. Then lift your hands until you are reaching as high as you can. While you are doing this, you can opt to lift your body until you are standing on your toes. Make sure that your spine is always flat on the wall. The whole cycle should last for four to six seconds. Some people think that this exercise is very easy but it can really be a bit more difficult since you need to always keep your spine flat against the wall.

*)With proper physical exercise, you will not only increase your chances of growing up to your fullest height potential but you will also be able to tone and strengthen your muscles and sustain a healthy and fit body.

Correct Your Body Posture

"Never slouch as doing so compresses the lungs, overcrowds other vital organs, rounds the back and throws you off balance."

- Joseph H. Pilates

When people wish to add extra inches to their height, the first things that come to their mind is to do specific lengthening exercises and boosting the levels of their growth hormones. These two options can really be effective in helping you grow taller yet a lot of people do not understand the importance of having good posture when they wish to enhance their height.

What you need to realize is that our spine is actually responsible for around 80 percent of our overall height. What this means is that if we are slouching or we do not aim to always be in good posture, we can actually be hampering our fullest height potential. However, the good news is that if you ever have bad posture now, it can be easily corrected. And when you make the effort to correct your posture, you can easily lengthen your spine and possibly add a couple of inches to your overall height.

There are still some people who are doubtful about this idea since they think that we stop growing taller after adolescence. But aiming to have good posture to increase your height is really effective because what you will be doing is really to get the most out of your height potential. You will not really be regenerating growth plates or things of that sort. A lot of people are actually around 2 inches shorter than their maximum potential height since their spines have become compressed due to bad posture. This just means that when they adjust their posture, they can lengthen their spine and add the missing inches.

How does this work?

As discussed above, our spine is accountable for more than 80 percent of our overall height. As we grow up, we acquire habits that lead to bad posture. We always look for "comfortable" positions while sitting or lying down without realizing that those comfy positions are actually bad for our posture. We commonly see young children carry heavy backpacks when going to school. This can actually lead to compressed spine. Even when you lean to one side when you stand up, you can actually throw your spine off and compress it which can make you shorter than how are supposed to be. But the good news is that you can actually get the lost inches back by focusing on improving your posture. This method is actually faster compared to other options.

What to Avoid

If you are looking for ways to improve your height, it is very essential for you to understand the things that need to be avoided because they can hinder your growth. Here are some techniques you can remember and avoid doing:

•Do not slouch while sitting down. You must have heard your mother say this to you a million of times already.

•Do not lie on your side. A lot of people have this habit of sleeping on their side without realizing that this is actually bad for their spine.

•Do not curl up in fetal position while sleeping. This position can compress your spine which could hinder it from growing to its highest potential.

•If you wish to carry backpacks and other bags, ensure that you do not fill them too heavily. As much as possible, carry your bags one at a time.

The above things that you need to avoid may seem simple but they can really help enhance your posture naturally. However, if you wish to achieve your fullest height potential, here are some of the things you can do:

•The most effective way to enhance your posture is to perform stretching exercises that focus on the spine. It is ideal to perform the stretches at least two times per day – first thing in the morning after you wake up and last thing at night before you sleep. But if your schedule will only allow you to do it once per day, that is alright as long as you do them religiously every day.

•You should be mindful of your posture while standing. A lot of people have weak back muscles and very tight chest muscle which makes their shoulders to slump forward. This posture can then lead to you hunching a little. In order to make sure that your posture is good while standing or walking, make sure that your shoulder blades are pinching together. Make sure that your shoulders are not rolling forward. If you want to check whether your posture is correct, you can hold two pencils – one in each hand and see if they are pointed straight ahead. If the pencils point to each other, you need to have your shoulders rolled back some more.

•Sleep on your back and do not use a pillow. I know a lot of people do not really like this technique especially when they are so used to sleeping on their sides and using pillows. But keep in mind that your body will eventually become used to this sleeping position and it will then feel normal to you. Sleeping with a pillow can put the upper part of your spine in an awkward position which can cause your head to tilt forward affecting your posture. Try sleeping on your back with no pillow even just for one week and you will see how your posture will improve and how better you will actually feel.

•When you sit down, make sure that your entire back is straight and flat against the chair. Make sure that both your shoulders are kept back. Imagine like you are attempting to crack an egg in the middle of your shoulder blades.

*)When you make the effort to correct your posture, you can easily lengthen your spine and possibly add a couple of inches to your overall height.

Get Adequate Sleep

"Sleeping is not time wasting."

- Mike Wilson

Our bodies grow when bone growth and cell division are stimulated by special hormones which are also called growth hormones. The growth hormones tell the muscles and bones in the skeleton to grow longer, bigger and stronger. For your growth hormones to function properly, it is important that you regularly get adequate sleep. The truth is that during the first two hours of sleep, your growth hormones start to spill out into your body system. When you do not have sufficient sleep, you are actually lowering the quantity of growth hormones that your body generates. Here are some useful tips that can help you in easily achieving deep level sleep:

•Make sure that you sleep in a dark room that is quiet and smells fresh. Exposing yourself to bright light while you sleep can actually trigger your brain to remain awake.

•Also make sure that the room where you sleep is properly ventilated because the quantity of clean air that is rich in oxygen can actually have an impact on your development.

•Sleep with comfortable, soft and clean clothes.

•Make sure that your feet and hands are warm while sleeping. Research studies have shown that keeping your feet and hands warm can aid in inducing deep sleep while cold feet and hands can stop you from getting into deep sleep.

•Regular exercise can help you get into deep sleep at night.

•A hot bath prior to sleeping can also aid in inducing deep sleep since it can relax your tense muscles and cleanse your body.

•Learn how to practice deep breathing and total relaxation. Do these techniques for a couple of minutes prior to sleeping.

•Make it a habit to sleep at the same time every day, even on weekends. This will allow your body to create a regular sleep rhythm. When sleeping at the same time has become a habit, your brain will automatically send your body "sleep signals" which can make you get into deep sleep faster and easier.

As discussed in the previous chapter, it is also important that you sleep with proper posture in order to stretch your spine and ultimately increase your height. Here are some useful tips that can help you sleep with proper posture:

•Make sure that your mattress is firm and comfortable. You can put a sheet of plywood below your mattress if you think that it is not firm enough. A firm mattress can help in aligning your spine in its natural position while you sleep. Because your spine will also be lengthened, the growth hormones can also easily travel to all parts of your body.

•While sleeping on your back, you can place a flat pillow underneath both of your knees in order to help your spine to align properly. This position can also prevent your back from aching and will allow your brain to absorb more blood rich in oxygen while you sleep.

•Avoid using high pillows can place strain on your back, shoulders and neck. High pillows can also lead to stunted growth because your spine will be arched while you sleep.

•Avoid sleeping with your face down to avoid straining your shoulders and neck and exaggerated swaybacks.

*)During deep sleep, your body generates the growth hormones that increase your height.

Avoid What Can Stunt Your Height Growth

"The only proper way to eliminate bad habits is to replace them with good ones."

- Jerome Hines

In the previous chapters, we have discussed the various techniques you can do to reach your maximum height potential. But aside from doing those techniques, it is also important for you to avoid certain things that can lead to stunted growth so that they will not cancel out the fruits of your efforts. Here are some of the things that you need to avoid:

Lack of Sleep

Perhaps this can be considered as the number one reason for stunted growth. As we have discussed in the previous chapter, it is during deep sleep when you actually grow in height since a huge quantity of growth hormones are generated and released at this time. When you have sleep deprivation, you are also preventing your body to generate the growth hormones that you need. Make sure that you sleep at least 7 to 8 hours every day.

Smoking Cigarettes

This is another leading cause for stunted growth. A research study has shown that young boys aged from 12 to 17 who smoke a minimum of ten cigarettes per day normally turn out to be one to two inches shorter compared to other boys of the same age who do not smoke. Smoking cigarettes can reduce the quantity of oxygen in your blood stream while increasing the amount of dangerous substances like carbon monoxide. When your body is oxygen deprived, your health is not only adversely affected but your growth can be stunted, as well. The nicotine from cigarettes can lead to narrowed blood vessels which can cause your body to not absorb enough nutrients to grow. Aside from this, you are also exposed to higher risks of lung cancer and heart attack.

Eating Too Much Carbs

You always need to keep in mind that carbohydrates are very essential in increasing height growth since they your body sufficient energy. But consuming a lot of carbs can lead to stunted growth since they can increase the level of insulin in your body which can prevent your body from efficiently utilizing the growth hormones. A lot of Asians consume a lot of carbs from corn and rice which is the reason why Asians have shorter average height compared to other nations who eat less carbs.

Drinking Soda

Soda drinks can lead to stunted growth primarily because of their carbonation that can deplete calcium from the bones in your body. With depleted calcium, you can experience lower bone density. Your body will also not be able to grow taller and stronger since the soda drinks are stealing the calcium that your bones need to grow. However, this does not mean that you should quit drinking soda altogether. Drinking them once in a while is okay. You just need to avoid drinking them in huge quantities on a regular basis. Avoid using soda as a substitute for water, especially when you are feeling thirsty.

*)It is important for you to avoid certain things that can lead to stunted growth so that they will not cancel out the fruits of your efforts.

How to Apply What You've Learned?

The techniques included in this book are not meant to be done in a sequential manner. You can actually start doing all of the techniques all at the same time. However, to make sure that you can effectively replace your old habit, it is ideal to focus on one goal at a time. After you have completed one goal, carry on to the next technique until you have developed good habits that can help you grow taller and healthier. Good luck!